Shattering the Food Pyramid

Dennis Karuri

Dennis Karuri

paraphrase any part, or the content within this book, without the consent of the author or publisher.

Disclaimer Notice:

Please note the information contained within this document is for educational and entertainment purposes only. All effort has been executed to present accurate, up to date, reliable, complete information. No warranties of any kind are declared or implied. Readers acknowledge that the author is not engaged in the rendering of legal, financial, medical or professional advice. The content within this book has been derived from various sources. Please consult a licensed professional before attempting any techniques outlined in this book.

By reading this document, the reader agrees that under no circumstances is the author responsible for any losses, direct or indirect, that are incurred as a result of the use of the information contained within this document, including, but not limited to, errors, omissions, or inaccuracies.

Dennis Karuri

Table of Contents

Introduction

If we really are what we eat, then it's not surprising that nutrition is so important. Creating a balanced diet is so important, that many governments have taken steps to provide information that is easy to understand and readily available. This is often found in the form of colorful graphics like food pyramids and food plates featuring different food groups and their suggested amounts or proportions.

However, these depictions are prone to flaws, some of which go all the way back to the very first pyramid, and they leave a lot of questions unanswered. Are those 2–3 recommended servings the same for an 80-pound child and a 180-pound adult? How much is in a serving? Can

Shattering the food pyramid

you eat steak, fruit salad, and baked potatoes every meal with bread as an appetizer since you include all the food groups? Butter counts as a serving of dairy, right?

The answer to all these questions can be found, but it's scattered across various sources, including buried deep on a couple of government-run websites. That's where this book comes in, providing answers to these questions and more in one convenient location.

The food pyramids have a long history and have been influenced by any number of factors over the years. Knowing how the food pyramids we see today came into being allows them to be utilized more effectively and sheds some light on the goals and intentions behind them.

Modern food pyramids and food plates, however, are primarily founded in nutrition research and the science behind how the body uses different kinds of food. A good foundation in these topics goes a long way towards being able to create a balanced diet that fits your needs.

This book helps you get that foundation by taking a closer look at what makes up the foods you eat and diving into what role things like protein, vitamins, and fats play in maintaining health.

With the rise of diet-related health concerns, understanding what goes into good nutrition is becoming increasingly important. Research has shown time and again that what we eat is closely related to our overall health, and certain parts of our diets hold greater sway over certain processes within our bodies than others. Too much of one nutrient or too little of another can have large repercussions, and there is a delicate interplay between many of the nutrients within the body.

Despite this seemingly endless complexity and intricacy, however, some simple generalizations can be made and adapted to an individual's needs. While there is no "one-size-fits-all" approach, you can define groups with shared characteristics to provide an approximation. These broader guidelines can then be modified and adapted to specific circumstances to provide the best fit.

This is accomplished by looking at nutrition at a very basic level, specifically at macronutrients and micronutrients, then applying the nutritional requirements to the food groups to drive decisions about how much of each is needed. While this book strives to provide more in-depth information than that provided on most graphics, it would be impossible to provide specific information for every reader's needs, and all recommendations listed should be considered in light of your age, gender, health status, and other relevant factors.

Chapter 1: Nutritional Foundation—Origin of the Food Pyramid

The food pyramid is one of the most recognizable symbols of a balanced diet and is commonly seen in elementary schools and pediatrician's offices to start creating healthy habits early in life. So, how did this colorful design come to represent the go-to nutritional guidance? What went into deciding how much of what group was best? Let's take a look into the history and origin of the food pyramid to find out.

Why the Food Pyramid

Was Designed

The first food 'pyramid' wasn't a pyramid–it was a circle. Originating in the US in 1943 during WWII, the Basic 7 was a diagram of seven groups of food recommended to eat each day, and it was heavily influenced by wartime shortages and rationing. This was readily adopted by many countries, though it wasn't the most nutritionally balanced depiction.

The next iteration, and the first true food pyramid, came from Sweden in the 1970s amidst soaring inflation and rapidly rising food prices. Sweden's National Board of Health and Welfare pulled from the Basic 7 grouping to divide foods into basic, which was essential in maintaining well-being, and supplementary, which filled in the vitamin and mineral gaps found in the basic foods. Although this provided a good foundation, it created a sense that supplementary foods could be excluded from the diet altogether, which would have resulted in various deficiencies.

To provide a better idea of an appropriately balanced diet, Anna Britt Agnsater, a member of the Swedish grocery cooperative, created a pyramid displaying the proportions of each group. This pyramid had three tiers: grains, legumes, potatoes, and milk on the bottom tier, fruits, vegetables, and juices in the middle, and meat, fish, and non-milk dairy products on the top.

From there, the food pyramid model was adopted in several countries. The overarching goal was to provide a quick visual guide to a balanced diet, and each country has implemented its own version of a food pyramid, though some have chosen other shapes to convey the information.

The United States began its process in 1992, and the end result, the Food Guide Pyramid, was less than perfect. Grains and cereals were recommended as the foundation of the diet with 6–11 servings per day. Dairy and meat were separated into their own groups with a recommended 2–3 servings each per day. Fruits and vegetables fell between dairy, meat, and grains with 2–5 servings recommended. Topping the pyramid were fats, oils, and sugars with the recommendation to use them sparingly.

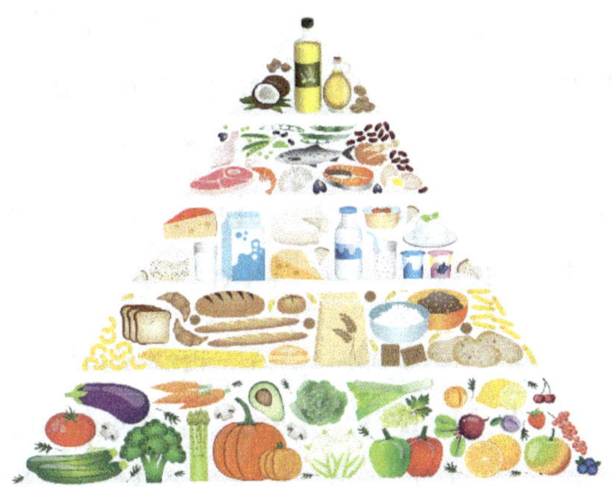

The Food Guide Pyramid was reviewed in 1995 when there was pressure from nutritionists to update the pyramid to support better health, but few significant changes were made. A true effort to shift the recommendations to a healthy diet began with the introduction of the MyPyramid in 2005, when the United States Department of Agriculture (USDA) switched the pyramid segments to the vertical plane, adjusted the proportions, and added steps to promote physical activity. While this was a step in the right direction, the vertical design made it more difficult to understand the relative proportions displayed, and it diverged from nutritionist recommendations.

In 2011, under the guidance of then-First Lady Michelle Obama, the pyramid was changed to a plate, called MyPlate, which shifted the focus from daily servings to relative proportions per meal. It emphasized fruits and vegetables over proteins and grains and reduced portion sizes.

The United Kingdom began working on its version of a food pyramid in 1994 with "The Balance of Good Health" model of nutrition, choosing to start with plate visualization. This depiction had a plate divided into five food groups based on suggested proportions, with the fruits and vegetables group and the grains group getting one-third of the plate each and the last third being divided between meats, dairy, and fats and oils.

In 2007, a newly named Eatwell plate was released with very few changes other than making it more appealing to the general public. This design was reviewed again in 2014 with an interest in addressing rising obesity and ensuring consistent messaging. New guidance recommended reducing sugar intake, including sugary drinks, and considered changes to recommendations for energy, iron, and fish suggested by the Scientific Advisory Committee on Nutrition (SACN).

Behind the Pyramid

Dennis Karuri

While both countries included specialists in their decision-making process, the US also allowed lobbyists, industry interests, and political goals to influence the final design. This significantly altered the original design submitted by a committee of nutritionists and worsened diet-related health problems over the years rather than improving them.

Most glaringly, the original recommendation for 5–9 servings of fresh fruits and vegetables to form the base was dropped down to 2–3 servings for each group per day, and the place of honor at the bottom of the pyramid was taken by grains and cereals at over the twice the original recommendation of 3–4 servings per day. There has been a shift towards more nutritionist recommended and scientifically-backed recommendations since 2005, but it's been a lengthy process to try to correct the original imbalance.

The UK started on the right foot, relying on evidence-based guidance from expert committees dedicated to nutrition. While they often review their Eatwell Plate and Eatwell Guide, the recommendations are only changed when there are changes to government dietary advice or significant publications reflecting new information.

The foundation for the US's MyPlate and the original, unadulterated food pyramid, and the UK's Balance of Good Health and Eatwell Plate is in nutritional science. However, our knowledge of nutrition keeps advancing, and the social and cultural aspects of each country create a unique lens which this information is viewed through.

Outside of official government depictions, researchers are incorporating the most current information to generate the most up-to-date graphics to inform the public. For instance, Harvard has designed their own food plate that replaces dairy with water and advocates limiting it to one to two servings, acknowledging that many cultures throughout history have thrived without dairy, as well as many people today who have chosen non-traditional diets.

The Harvard food plate also includes healthy oils in its depiction, advocating for moderation over elimination and emphasizing that the type of fat included is just as important as the amount.

Shattering the food pyramid

Similar discussions are going on around the long-standing recommendation to lower sodium to reduce the incidence of high blood pressure and promote heart health. Ongoing research has found no evidence to support this claim, and as more information comes to light, this recommendation may fall to the wayside after its more than 50 years of inclusion in dietary guidelines.

As nutritional science advances, the recommendations seen in food pyramids will likely shift accordingly. Using all available information allows for the most accurate suggestions to be made, and incorporating discoveries about previously held beliefs about what's healthy and what isn't will provide the best guidance to be available.

How to Use the Food Pyramid

The food pyramid is meant as general guidance for the majority of the population. That said, it's not perfect, and it shouldn't be taken as an absolute. Instead, the food pyramid is a reminder to include a variety of foods in your overall diet. It can provide a baseline for relative proportions that can be adjusted to individual needs and preferences. It emphasizes moderation in all things and focuses on fresh whole foods instead of overly processed foods with little nutritional value.

Children under two have different nutritional needs, and the food pyramid should only be a target for children as they approach five years old. A pediatrician should be included in the discussion about diets for very young children to support the needs of their rapidly growing bodies.

Additionally, those with various medical conditions might have nutritional needs that are vastly different from the recommendations in the food pyramid. These individuals should also consult with their physician to see what kind of diet would be best for their personal needs. Though you may have been taught the food pyramid as a child, it isn't meant for all situations.

Where the Food Pyramid Falls Short

The food pyramid has several flaws and drawbacks, though there have been steps taken to correct some of them. The biggest flaw, and its greatest appeal, is its simplicity. A simple graphic is very easy for people to read and remember, but it's also very prone to misunderstanding and confusion, especially if there isn't good labeling.

Shattering the food pyramid

Many depictions of the food pyramid only have labels for the groups with a brief description at the bottom, and the rest is left to the imagination.

The US's first food pyramid was especially hindered by this flaw, along with the previously mentioned shortcomings. The fats, oils, and sweets group was represented by white and yellow dots that were also sprinkled throughout all the other segments, not just the one at the top. This gave the impression that they weren't important when they were included with food from one of the other groups, and led to rampant over-consumption of the group that was supposed to be kept to a minimum.

This lack of clarity leads to the next flaw: the lack of distinction between types of foods in a group. The processing of many foods and ingredients leaches several of the nutrients from the final product. This is why we have things like fortified milk and enriched flours and bread, to make up for what's missing and prevent deficiencies when eating staple foods.

Because of this, it's important to focus on including whole foods and minimally processed ingredients whenever possible. Unfortunately, the examples shown on many food pyramids are easily recognized processed foods, lending themselves to the belief that processed foods are just as healthy as whole foods and can make up a large part of a balanced diet. Similarly, it doesn't mention that some types of fat and oil are healthier than others, resulting in higher levels of saturated relative to

Shattering the food pyramid

unsaturated fats being included in the diet.

Yet another flaw is the shape itself. Organizing the food groups in a pyramid, in theory, seems like a great way of showing the hierarchy of which foods should be consumed more or less than the others. The bigger the segment, the more of that food you should eat. However, the way people tend to read top to bottom and interpret what they see first as the most important.

This has led to an overemphasis on fats, oils, and sweets, the food group displayed at the very top. It's also hard for people to recognize that what's on the bottom is the most important, even though it's intended to be the biggest segment. Rotating the segments so they're vertical does little to improve this and can make it even more difficult to see which groups are supposed to be more important.

Finally, one of the more frustrating aspects of the food pyramid is that it's very generic. While this is great to provide a starting point, many people don't realize that it should be customized to their individual needs, or even how to use the ranges provided in the illustration. These guidelines shouldn't try to cater exactly to every person that might see them, but they should at least offer different recommendations based on categories such as age and activity level to provide a better understanding of what each group might need.

Creating a Balanced Diet

Shattering the food pyramid

Despite all the issues food pyramids have, the goal of helping people ensure adequate nutrition to promote health is a noble one. While individualized diet recommendations are beyond the scope of this book, some general suggestions for creating a balanced diet can be made before we dive deeper into macronutrients, micronutrients, and food groups.

The concept of including different food groups allows for variety and makes it easier to get all the macronutrients and micronutrients needed without additional supplements. You should also look at what kinds of foods within each group you're eating. Prioritize whole foods and fresh ingredients whenever possible, and try to incorporate more unsaturated fats than saturated fats. Remember to use moderation in everything, and aim for balancing your diet over a day or a week rather than each meal.

As far as improving the food pyramid goes, the switch to a food plate is a step in the right direction. Each food group should have a label indicating how much of the diet it should make up. All of the recommendations should be firmly backed by science without the influence of politics or industry lobbying. If possible, additional material such as pamphlets and longer guidebooks should be available to explain the food plate in more detail and provide more specific information for different ages, activity levels, and similar designations.

(If you want to get into the nitty-gritty details of how humans view graphics, a bar graph or column chart would be a

Shattering the food pyramid

better idea since humans aren't that great at comparing areas. A food plate is more appealing, though, and adding the right labels can overcome this hurdle.)

Chapter 2: The Basics—Macronutrients

Nutrition is a complex and ever-growing topic best broken into smaller pieces for discussion. Let's start with macronutrients.

What Is a Macronutrient?

Macronutrients consist of proteins, carbohydrates, and lipids, a term used interchangeably with fat, which are needed in higher quantities than micronutrients. Each of these serves its own function in the body, and you need them all in different proportions for optimal health and well-being. Deficiencies of macronutrients are less common than excesses in most developed countries, but it's still important to avoid restricting them unnecessarily.

Carbohydrates are variably sized molecules that are defined by their set ratio of one carbon atom to every two hydrogen atoms to every one oxygen atom. They can be divided into groups of monosaccharides, disaccharides, and polysaccharides based on the number of carbons they have.

Monosaccharides have one six-carbon group typically arranged in a ring. Of the monosaccharides, the most important one is glucose. Glucose is the body's primary energy source, and many cells, including neurons in the brain and many immune cells, can only use glucose to generate their energy. Glucose has two different isomers, L-glucose and D-glucose. The isomer used by humans is D-glucose, also known as dextrose.

Other monosaccharides are fructose and galactose. Fructose is often used as a sweetener in processed foods, but it doesn't have the same functions as glucose. Galactose can be converted into glucose to be better utilized by the body.

Disaccharides are pairs of monosaccharides linked together. These include sucrose, maltose, and lactose. Maltose is made of two glucose molecules while sucrose contains glucose and fructose. Lactose is made of galactose and glucose and is the main sugar in animal milk.

Polysaccharides are much longer chains of monosaccharides and are often referred to as complex carbohydrates because they have more parts than mono- and di-saccharides, which are often called simple sugars. Polysaccharides are broken down into mono- and di-saccharides to be absorbed from the intestines.

There are three main types of polysaccharides: starch, glycogen, and cellulose. Glycogen is formed from long, branching chains of glucose and is very hydrophilic, requiring large amounts of water to be stored. Starch has various monosaccharides strung together and is broken down into smaller pieces by the same enzymes that break down the disaccharides.

Cellulose is a structural polysaccharide found in plants and is responsible for the rigidity of stalks and stems as well as the outer coverings of seeds. Humans are unable to break down cellulose at the molecular level because we don't produce the required enzymes. However, cellulose still plays an important role in the human body and is a necessary nutrient, often referred to as dietary fiber.

One final class of carbohydrates is oligosaccharides, a subcategory of polysaccharides. They are made from two to ten simple sugars and are poorly digestible. Like cellulose, they still serve a purpose within the digestive tract, and their potential benefits are the subject of ongoing research.

Proteins are formed from long chains of molecules called amino acids, which consist of an amino group, an acid group, and one of 20 unique side chains. The side chains determine the overall structure of an amino acid as well as its charge and function within the protein.

The amino acids are as follows:

- histidine
- glycine
- leucine
- isoleucine
- tyrosine
- methionine
- threonine
- serine

- arginine
- lysine
- taurine
- phenylalanine
- cysteine
- serine
- tryptophan
- valine
- glutamine
- asparagine
- aspartate
- glutamate

Of these 20, 11 of them can be synthesized in the body, and nine of them, called essential amino acids, must be included since the body has no way of making them when needed.

Shattering the food pyramid

Proteins can be anywhere from less than 20 to over 50 amino acids long, and their structure and function are determined by both the number and types of amino acids present, which represents the first level of structure of proteins. The next level of structure is in what locations the protein will bend, fold, and twist itself. This is driven by the size and charge of the amino acid side chains and where they are in relation to others.

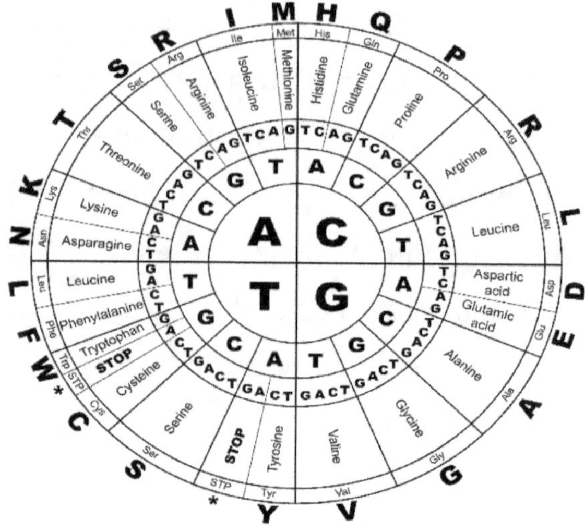

These folds and twists are referred to as alpha helices and beta sheets, and the three-dimensional shape they create is the third level of structure. When multiple of these folded chains of amino acids, called polypeptides, come together, they form the fourth level of structure that is often required for them to function properly.

The order of amino acids for each protein is encoded in DNA. Because every plant and animal species has different DNA, they all produce different proteins and have different ratios of amino acids. Proteins are also one of the molecules recognized by the immune system, and the difference in the proteins produced by humans and those produced by plants and animals is one of the contributors to allergies.

Since much of the structure of proteins is determined by non-covalent bonds within alpha helices and beta sheets and between different polypeptides, they require certain pH and temperature conditions to retain their structure and function.

When the temperature and pH vary too far from normal, physiologic conditions, the proteins undergo a process called denaturing, where the non-covalent bonds begin to come apart and the protein reverts to a linear line of amino acids. We take advantage of this process to a certain extent when cooking foods, and it's a key part of protein digestion.

Lipids come in many different varieties and fulfill many different functions. They are typically hydrophobic compounds and are generally divided into triglycerides, phospholipids, and glycolipids, which are made of fatty acids bound to another molecule. Cholesterols act as their own category without fatty acids and have a ring structure instead of straight chains like other forms of lipid.

Fatty acids are classified by the number of double bonds in their chemical structure and are broken down into saturated, unsaturated, and trans fatty acids. Saturated fatty acids have no double bonds between the carbon atoms, giving them the maximum number of hydrogen atoms. These fatty acids pack together more closely and are more often found as solids at room temperature.

Unsaturated fatty acids have one or more double bonds between carbon atoms, creating a kinked structure rather than a linear one. This prevents them from effectively stacking, and they are more often found as liquids at room temperature.

Trans fatty acids are unsaturated fatty acids that have undergone hydrogenation to improve stability and shelf life. These are typically considered unhealthy, and many food producers have begun to reduce the number of trans fats.

Phospholipids are two fatty acids bound to a phosphate group. The phosphate end is hydrophilic while the fatty acids are hydrophobic, making phospholipids amphipathic. Triglycerides are three fatty acids bound to a glycerol molecule. The fatty acids are removed and replaced using esterification reactions to create a variety of different triglycerides to be used throughout the body.

Macronutrients in the Diet

Shattering the food pyramid

While we often treat the food groups as distinct and separate, almost all foods have some level of all three macronutrients, with the notable exceptions of meats, which contain little to no carbohydrates, and oils, which contain no protein or carbohydrates. This prevalence allows for many different kinds of diets, such as dairy-free or vegan, without major macronutrient deficiencies, though care must still be taken to balance other nutrients in the diet.

Though macronutrients are relatively ubiquitous to most food groups, some have higher concentrations than others. Meats, for example, contain high levels of protein, and grains contain high levels of carbohydrates. Many types of nuts are also high in protein. Fruits tend to have moderate levels of natural sugars, and some vegetables contain high levels of starch, both of which fall into the carbohydrates category. Dairy products can also have relatively high levels of fat and protein, though this can be drastically altered by processing and varies greatly from product to product.

When looking at protein in the diet, the constituent amino acids should be considered. While the body can make the majority of amino acids, tryptophan, valine, histidine, leucine, lysine, isoleucine, threonine, methionine, and phenylalanine must be included in the diet.

Lipids can be found in every food group in small amounts, though they are predominantly found in foods from the fats and oils group. Meats and dairy have variable amounts of fat, and in many instances can contribute significantly to your level of fat consumption. Fruits and vegetables have very low levels of fat and no cholesterol. Grains have low levels of fat on their own, though many of the foods in the grains category also include ingredients from other food groups that can increase the fat content.

How the Body Uses Macronutrients

Macronutrients are the main drivers of caloric intake in the diet and are used as energy sources by the body, though carbohydrates serve this function much more than the other two. Proteins and carbohydrates both provide roughly four calories per gram (g) while fats provide roughly nine calories per g. One thing to keep in mind here is that while the term 'calories' is often used in conversations about nutrition, what is actually being discussed are kilocalories (kcals). A kcal is 1,000 calories as measured by a calorimeter and is sometimes written as Calories in scientific publications. While this rarely becomes relevant when reading food labels or using calorie-tracking tools, it becomes an important distinction in some research articles and can be misleading if not accounted for.

Carbohydrates provide the vast majority of the energy in the body since their most basic components are simple sugars. Fats are the way the body stores its excess energy, but they require more steps to be usable by cells and serve other functions besides providing energy. Similarly, while proteins can be used to provide energy when no other sources are available, they are much more valuable broken down and recycled into new proteins.

While carbohydrates are the primary source of energy, typically in the form of glucose, their hydrophilic nature makes them unsuitable for being stored in large amounts. They require large amounts of water and take more space to store less energy relative to fat. The body only stores enough glycogen to provide approximately one day's worth of energy, and the rest is converted into fat.

Macronutrients are also the body's primary building blocks and the divers of every reaction within the body. Proteins are used to create everything from muscles and connective tissue to hormones to enzymes that catalyze chemical reactions. They are found in cell membranes, within the intracellular fluid, and in the extracellular and interstitial spaces. They are responsible for the breakdown of nutrients in the GI tract, help copy DNA during cell division, and convert glucose and fats to ATP, the usable form of energy within the body. A protein called hemoglobin is responsible for delivering oxygen to all the tissues, which is essential for normal functioning.

Proteins are also responsible for regulating many processes and levels throughout the body. Insulin and ghrelin are all protein hormones that regulate blood glucose, hunger, and the levels of micronutrients. Many neurotransmitters like serotonin and dopamine are also proteins. Proteins can even regulate their own production through feedback systems that inhibit or promote the enzymes involved in their synthesis reactions.

Lipids are just as pervasive throughout the body as proteins and are key in many signaling pathways. Cell membranes are made of a bilayer of phospholipids interspersed with cholesterol and transport proteins. The phospholipids are arranged with their hydrophobic fatty acid tails facing toward each other and their hydrophilic phosphate heads facing away from each other, creating a semi-permeable membrane that separates the intracellular and extracellular spaces.

Triglycerides and cholesterols can also be found in cell membranes to help influence their fluidity. Cholesterol is also a steroid hormone that can be used to produce other hormones like testosterone, estrogen, and progesterone. Cholesterol and its derivatives act as signaling molecules throughout the body.

Unbound fatty acids are another group of signaling molecules. They most commonly act as inflammatory mediators and are produced by the cyclooxygenase pathway. This pathway is what is targeted by non-steroidal anti-inflammatories (NSAIDs) like ibuprofen and acetaminophen. These signaling molecules are also important in maintaining the health and mucosal surfaces like those lining the stomach and intestines, and a lack of proper production due to disease or over-use of NSAIDs can result in mucosal damage and bleeding into the GI tract.

Macronutrient Requirements

While many things can impact macronutrient requirements, especially as they relate to energy needs, there are a few general guidelines that can be adjusted to meet your individual needs.

Generally speaking, adults should consume approximately 0.75 g of protein per day for every kilogram (kg) of body weight. This equates to roughly 55 g per day for the average man and 45 g per day for the average woman. Women who are pregnant have an increased need for all nutrients, including protein, and should consume roughly 70 g of protein per day. These numbers should be moved up or down as appropriate for your weight to ensure you aren't getting too much or too little.

Children from 4 to 10 years old should be getting up to 29 g per day of protein to support their growing bodies. Children and teens over 10 and under 19 should be consuming from 45 g of protein up to 58 g to support their continued growth and account for any metabolic changes caused by puberty.

The recommended daily amount of carbohydrates for average adults is approximately 30–50% of your daily energy intake, which varies based on your energy needs. While many fad diets emphasize reducing carbs to lose weight, they cannot be cut completely from the diet or reduced too drastically and must be included at a minimum level to ensure overall health. However, they should not be consumed in excess, either, and reducing carbohydrates can be beneficial in situations of overconsumption.

Fats should be consumed in the smallest amounts of all the macronutrients. Within that amount, different types of fats should be consumed in different amounts to support various functions throughout the body. These types will be discussed in more detail in the chapter discussing their primary food group. Overall, though, fats should be balanced among the different types and confined to only 20–35% of your daily energy intake to avoid issues related to excessive fat in the diet.

Chapter 3: The Basics— Micronutrients

Next on the list, and finishing off the more basic topics, is micronutrients. Once we understand these, we can move on to the food groups and how they interact with macronutrients and micronutrients.

What Is a Micronutrient?

Micronutrients are needed in small amounts and are vital to a wide variety of functions throughout the body. They consist of vitamins, which are organic molecules that are sensitive to heat and processing, and minerals, hardy, inorganic compounds with a variety of functions. These two nutrients are also categorized even further.

Vitamins are broken down into water-soluble and fat-soluble. Water-soluble vitamins are vitamin C (ascorbic acid) and the vitamin B complex. The vitamin B complex includes the following:

- thiamine (b1)

- riboflavin (b2)

- niacin (b3)

- pantothenic acid (b5)

- pyridoxine (b6)

- biotin (b7)

- folate (b9)

- cobalamin (b12)

Water-soluble vitamins are found in very limited amounts in the body and must be included in the diet every day to prevent deficiencies.

Fat-soluble vitamins are vitamin A (retinol and beta-carotene), vitamin D (calcitriol, ergocalciferol (D2), and cholecalciferol (D3)), vitamin E (tocopherol), and vitamin K. Because fat deposits exist throughout the body, fat-soluble vitamins can be stored in great amounts and released as needed. Deficiencies of these are rare outside of incredibly restrictive or unbalanced diets, general malnourishment, and intestinal disease or injury preventing appropriate absorption. Excesses are more common, especially with the prevalence of over-the-counter

Shattering the food pyramid

supplements, and result in toxic effects throughout the body.

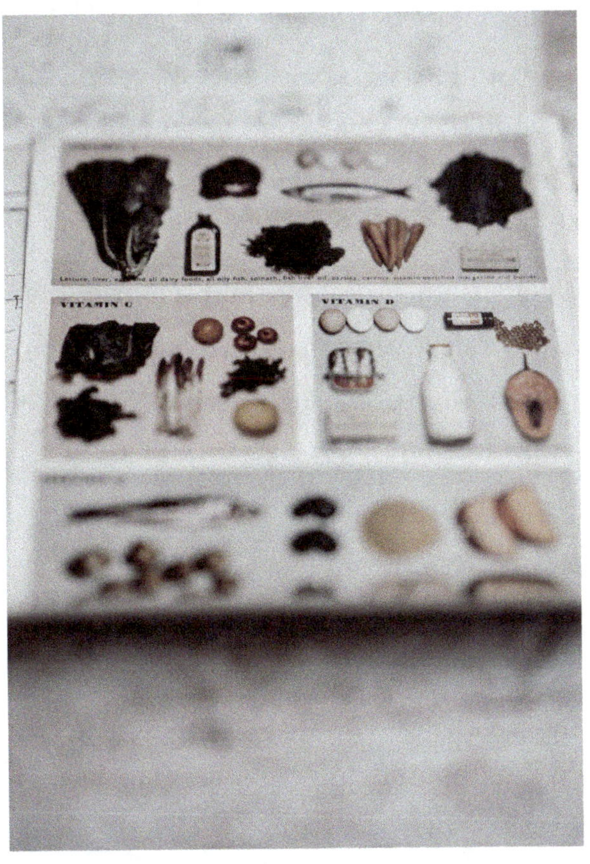

Minerals are broken down into macrominerals and microminerals, or trace minerals. Macrominerals are needed in the largest amounts and include calcium, magnesium, phosphorus, sulfur, manganese, and potassium. Trace minerals are only required in small amounts by the body and include iron, zinc, copper, selenium, iodine, sodium, and chloride. Potassium, sodium, and chloride are also referred to as electrolytes and are often discussed together due to their interrelated functions.

Micronutrients in the Diet

Vitamins and minerals are found in a variety of foods, though certain foods contain higher amounts of a given micronutrient than others. Vitamins are found in both animal and plant foods.

Fat-soluble vitamins are found in the parts of foods with higher fat content, while water-soluble vitamins are found in foods with high water contents like fruits.

Two vitamins are unique in the way they are obtained and processed by the body. Vitamin D is consumed in an inactive form and must be activated by sunlight in the cells of the skin. Vitamin K can be produced by bacteria in the gastrointestinal system at significant levels, up to 75% of the required daily amount.

Many minerals are found predominantly in animal products, and those that are found in plants are found in most green vegetables, legumes, bananas, and nuts. Sodium and chloride are especially abundant in table salt. They are also found in many fortified foods, such as iodine in iodized salt and iron in enriched flour and bread.

While macronutrients are found almost exclusively in foods, many microminerals can also be found in over-the-counter or prescription supplements designed to fill in the gaps in your diet or to provide additional amounts to compensate for increased requirements due to illness, injury, or pregnancy. Over-the-counter supplements that are referred to as "multi-vitamins" often contain water-soluble vitamins and trace minerals, as well as fat-soluble vitamins and macrominerals that aren't as prevalent in common foods, and are designed to cover a wide variety of needs. You can also find over-the-counter supplements that only contain one micronutrient to cover a specific dietary deficiency or increased need.

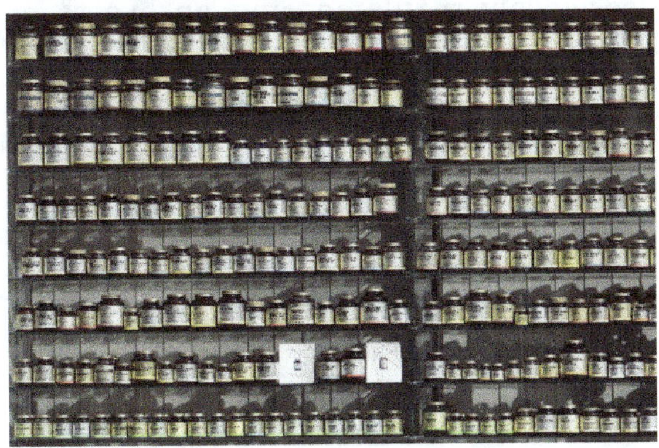

How the Body Uses Micronutrients

Micronutrients have a role in almost every function in the body. They act as cofactors for enzymes, help the movement of nutrients into cells and waste products out, enable the generation of enzymes, support healthy bones, skin, and hair, and more. They are closely regulated, and an excess or deficiency of any of these can throw the body into chaos.

Vitamin A protects the integrity of the retina and aids in the development of the different cell types found circulating in the blood. Vitamin D is involved in the absorption of calcium and maintaining its balance with phosphorus as well as influencing the strength of bone.

Vitamin E is an antioxidant that works in combination with selenium to protect cells from free radicals and helps to prevent degenerative diseases that lead to cognitive dysfunction. Vitamin K is a versatile compound that is predominantly responsible for the activation of the coagulation cascade in response to injury.

The vitamin B complex is crucial for metabolism and energy levels, especially thiamin and riboflavin, and for maintaining nerves and cognitive function. Vitamin C is well-known for its role in preventing diseases like scurvy, contributes to many enzyme-driven reactions within the body, and assists the immune system in getting rid of bacteria, viruses, and debris from cell turnover.

Calcium plays a huge role in the musculoskeletal system. It's required for skeletal, smooth, and heart muscles to be able to contract, and it's an essential component of bone that allows for structure and rigidity. Phosphorus is another key element in ensuring the strength of bone as well as driving energy and protein production.

Sulfur is used to create certain amino acids, the building blocks of protein, and helps maintain pH in the bloodstream. Magnesium is involved in nerve conduction and muscle conduction. Zinc helps reduce inflammation and aids in proper digestion and absorption of nutrients. Copper is used to make red blood cells and connective tissues as well as to aid in the absorption of iron.

Selenium is an antioxidant that works synergistically with vitamin E and is essential for muscle growth and development. Iodine is used to produce thyroid hormones which in turn drive many metabolic processes. Manganese is yet another element involved in the maintenance of bones and works in conjunction with vitamin A in the coagulation cascade. Iron is part of hemoglobin and carries oxygen through the bloodstream to all parts of the body.

The electrolytes, sodium, potassium, and chloride help maintain hydration status within the cells and balance the body's pH. Sodium and potassium act together to move larger molecules in and out of the cell as well as help with energy production. Sodium is required in the diet to allow for appropriate absorption of glucose in the GI tract, and potassium performs a vital role in the electrical conduction required for muscle contraction.

Micronutrient Requirements

The requirements of different micronutrients depend on the bioavailability of a given vitamin or mineral from a given food or supplement. For minerals, bioavailability can be impacted by what other minerals are present and in what ratios. For example, calcium and phosphorus compete for absorption sites, so a diet high in phosphorus inhibits calcium absorption and vice versa. For vitamins, the bioavailability can be impacted by whether they come from a natural source or were synthesized in a lab.

Recommended amounts for vitamins and minerals are often reported in milligrams (mg), micrograms (mcg), and international units (IU). These units can be converted back and forth, and there is

Shattering the food pyramid

occasional inconsistency in which units are used on food and supplement labels.

For natural sources, general vitamin recommendations for men are as follows:

- Vitamin A-900 to 3,000 mcg (≈3,000 to 10,000 IU)

- Vitamin C-90 to 2,000 mg

- Vitamin D-15 to 50 mcg (≈600 to 2,000 IU)

- Vitamin E-15 to 1,000 mg (≈22 to 1,500 IU)

- Vitamin K-120 mcg

- Thiamin-1.2 mg

- Folate-400 to 1,000 mcg

- Niacin-16 mg

- Riboflavin-1.3 mg

- Pyridoxine (B6)-1.3 to 100 mg

- Biotin-30 mcg

- Pantothenic Acid-5 mg

- Cobalamin (B12)-2.4 mcg

Vitamin E and folate have significantly different bioavailabilities when synthetically made. Synthetic vitamin E has a lower bioavailability, resulting in a recommended amount of 30 IU per day. Folic acid, the synthetic form of folate, has higher bioavailability, and the recommended amount per day is 400 mcg of a Daily Folate Equivalent (DFE). A DFE of folic acid is roughly 0.6 mcg when taken with food or 0.5 mcg when taken on an empty stomach.

The daily mineral recommendations for men are listed below:

- Calcium-1,300 to 2,000 mg

- Magnesium-420 mg

Shattering the food pyramid

- Phosphorus-1,250 to 4,000 mg

- Iron-8 to 45 mg

- Zinc-11 to 40 mg

- Copper-900 to 10,000 mcg

- Selenium-55 to 400 mcg

- Iodine-150 to 1,100 mcg

- Manganese-2.3 to 11 mg

- Sodium-2,300 mg

- Chloride-2,300 mg

- Potassium-4,700 mg

For natural sources, general vitamin recommendations for women are as follows:

- Vitamin A-700 to 3,000 mcg (≈2,333 to 10,000 IU)

- Vitamin C-75 to 2,000 mg

- Vitamin D-15 to 50 mcg ($\approx$600 to 2,000 IU)

- Vitamin E-15 to 1,000 mg ($\approx$22 to 1,5000 IU)

- Vitamin K-90 mcg

- Thiamin-1.1 mg

- Folate-400 to 1,000 mcg

- Niacin-14 mg

- Riboflavin-1.1 mg

- Pyridoxine (B6)-1.3 to 100 mg

- Biotin-30 mcg

- Pantothenic Acid-5 mg

- Cobalamin (B12)-2.4 mcg

Synthetic vitamin E has a recommended amount of 30 IU per day. The recommended amount of folic acid per day is 400 mcg of a DFE.

Shattering the food pyramid

The daily mineral recommendations for women are listed below:

- Calcium-1,300 to 2,000 mg

- Magnesium-320 mg

- Phosphorus-1,250 to 4,000 mg

- Iron-18 to 45 mg

- Zinc-8 to 40 mg

- Copper-900 to 10,000 mcg

- Selenium-55 to 400 mcg

- Iodine-150 to 1,100mcg

- Manganese-1.8 to 11 mg

- Sodium-2,300 mg

- Chloride-2,300 mg

- Potassium-4,700 mg

Because sulfur is found in over 1% of the amino acids found in proteins, it doesn't have known specific requirements, and diets with adequate amounts of protein also provide sufficient amounts of sulfur.

Recommendations for children are more variable due to their fluctuating growth rates. However, all the micronutrients should be included in children's diets and be gradually increased to the levels for adults as they mature. Consult with your child's pediatrician for more definitive recommendations to ensure they're getting adequate nutrition and growing appropriately for their age.

Chapter 4: Food Groups—Grains, Fats, and Oils

The grains food group and the fats and oils food groups are major drivers of calorie intake in the diet. They also provide a handful of other essential nutrients, though neither can provide a balanced diet either alone or when combined. These are also the food groups most often targeted by diets promoting weight loss, and the grains food group is the center of discussion in gluten-free diets.

Dennis Karuri

What's in the Grain Food Group?

Grains, also called cereals or cereal grains, are a class of foods made from wheat, rice, oats, barley, and cornmeal. This group includes things like bread, oatmeal, pasta, and tortillas, and can be further broken down into whole grains and refined grains.

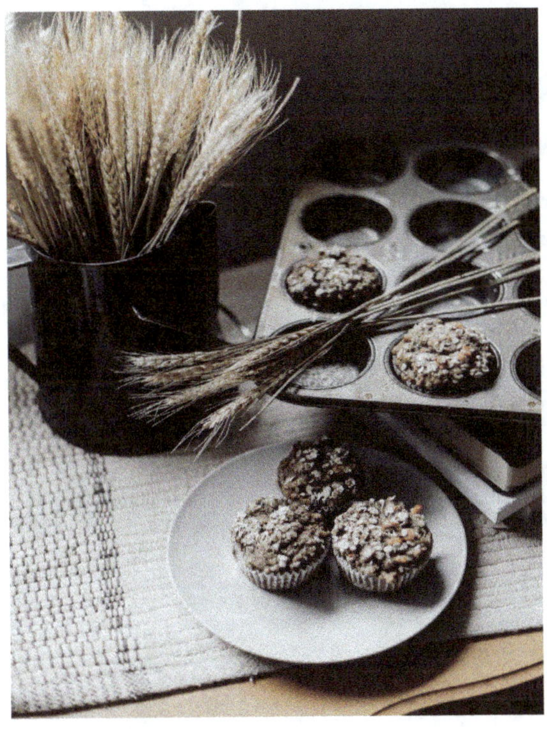

Whole grains contain the whole kernel, including the bran, endosperm, and germ. Refined grains are processed into fine flour or meal, and the germ and bran are separated from the endosperm. Refined grains should be enriched to replace the vitamins and minerals removed with the bran and germ. The dietary fiber lost during processing is not replaced during enrichment. Foods advertised as whole grain should be made with 100% whole grains, and some foods are made with a mixture of refined and whole grains.

What's in the Fats and Oils Food Group?

Oils and fats are naturally found as parts of other foods. The primary difference between fats and oils is whether they are liquid or solid at room temperature. This is determined by the underlying chemical structure of the specific kinds of fat making up a given product, and there are three general classes of fats influencing this, though there are also other types of fat.

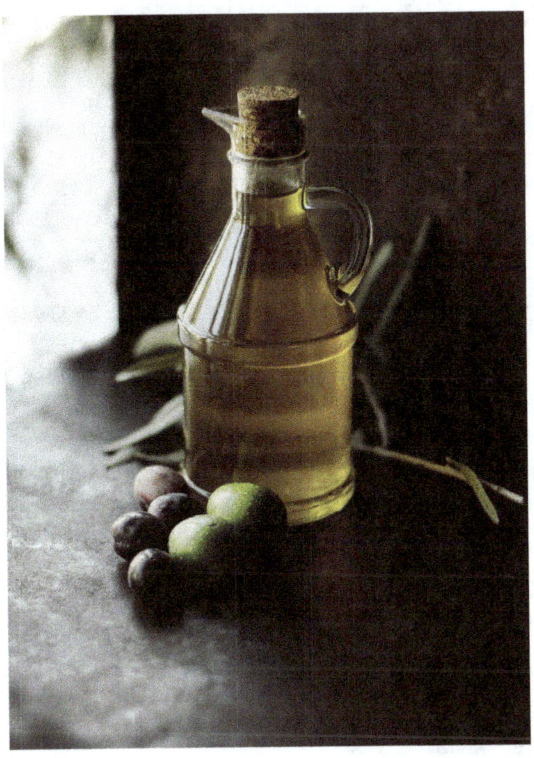

The fats and oils found within plant and animal foods can be processed and removed to make stand-alone products like margarine, olive oil, and fish oils. These can then be used to cook with, such as when frying or sauteing dishes, or as ingredients in other prepared foods like baked goods and dressings. It's important to remember that these fats exist—as well as what kind of fats they are—when trying to create a balanced diet.

Some products that are referred to as oils don't actually fall into the oils category. These include things like coconut oil and palm oil that are solid at room temperature. Nutritionally speaking, they are more comparable to solid fats like butter and shortening due to their saturated fat content relative to other oils.

High—Density Nutrients in the Grain Food Group

Grains can contain any number of nutrients, especially whole grains. The kind and amounts of nutrients can depend a lot on the type of soil they're grown in, what kinds of fertilizers, if any, are used, and environmental conditions such as droughts and early freezes. All grains, however, contain a significant amount of carbohydrates and often serve as their primary source in the diet.

In addition to carbohydrates, grains can contain high levels of dietary fiber. While dietary fiber doesn't offer nutritive value to the body, which is why it wasn't discussed above, it promotes GI health and aids in digestion and absorption of other nutrients by slowing down the movement of food through the intestines.

Whole grains are good sources of riboflavin, folate, niacin, and thiamin along with minerals such as iron, magnesium, and selenium. The selenium content is directly related to the soil the grains are grown in, with grains grown in high-selenium soil having higher levels and grains grown in selenium-deficient soil having lower levels.

Since most of these micronutrients are contained within the germ and bran, they must be added back to refined grains. The vitamins riboflavin, niacin, and thiamin are added back to refined grains, as well as iron since they are both vital to health and needed in larger amounts than folate, selenium, and magnesium.

Grains are considered a staple food, though they may take on different forms in different cultures. Their traditional prevalence in many people's diets is a large part of the reason refined grains are often required to be enriched by governing bodies. The loss of micronutrients during processing could quickly lead to deficiencies if they weren't found in sufficient quantities in other parts of the diet.

High—Density Nutrients in the Fats and Oils Food Group

In addition to being a source of abundant energy, more than twice that found in proteins and carbohydrates, the fats and oils food group is also the primary source of fatty acids. Fatty acids are a specific portion of fats that can exist on their own or as part of other lipids (fat) compounds such as phospholipids or triglycerides. They also determine whether fats are considered saturated or unsaturated.

These fatty acids drive many processes within the body, including inflammatory cascades and forming cell membranes, and are an important precursor for many hormones. The vast majority of these fatty acids can be made from other fats in the human body, but one essential fatty acid, called Omega-3 fatty acid, cannot be produced by the human body and must be included in the diet.

While fat molecules themselves may not include many micronutrients, fatty foods and oils are a good source of the fat-soluble vitamins A, D, E, and K. Fats are also essential to the proper absorption of these vitamins even if they come from other sources, such as vegetables.

Recommendations for Grains

Recommendations for grains are listed in ounce-equivalents (oz-equiv). An oz-equiv is how much of a finished product contains one ounce's worth of grain. Some examples of common foods are one slice of bread, one six-inch tortilla, and three cups of popped popcorn. To approximate the needs of different groups, recommendations are divided by age and gender. No matter which recommendations match your needs best, at least half of all grains in the diet should be whole grains.

Toddlers aged 1 to 2 years old should have 1.75 to 3 oz-equiv per day in their diet. Children between 2 and 4 years old should have 3 to 5 oz-equiv per day, and children from 5 to 8 should have 4 to 6 oz-equiv per day. For nine years and older, recommendations diverge between males and females.

Girls between 9 and 13 years old should have 5 to 7 oz-equiv per day, and between 14 and 18 years old, they should have 6 to 8 oz-equiv per day. Women should continue consuming 6 to 8 oz-equiv per day from 19 to 30 years old, then decrease to 5 to 7 oz-equiv per day from 31 onward.

Boys between 9 and 13 years old should have 5 to 9 oz-equiv per day, and boys from 14 to 18 years old should have 6 to 10 oz-equiv per day. Men should increase to 8 to 10 oz-equiv per day from 19 to 30 years old, then decrease slightly to 7 to 10 oz-equiv per day between 31 and 59, and decrease again to 6 to 9 oz-equiv per day from age 60 onward.

Since grains are high in carbohydrates, one of the body's primary sources of energy, as well as B complex vitamins, individual needs can vary greatly based on things that impact energy needs like activity level, and for women, their pregnancy and lactation status. Grains, like all foods, should be eaten in moderation.

Dennis Karuri

Recommendations for Oils and Fats

Recommendations for fat are less specific. They typically use the percent of daily energy intake as a unit of measurement and often focus on the kinds of fat consumed. Research on the value of fats is constantly evolving, leading to continually updated recommendations.

At the time of this writing, it is recommended that total fat consumption not exceed 35% of daily calorie intake, though higher fat diets may be appropriate for some individuals. This should consist predominantly of unsaturated fats, especially polyunsaturated fats and those containing higher levels of omega-3 fatty acids. Saturated fats should be limited to no more than 7% of daily calorie intake, though there is insufficient evidence of saturated fats increasing the risk of heart disease to support removing them from the diet entirely. Any saturated fats removed from the diet should be replaced with either unsaturated fats or complex carbohydrates rather than simple sugars. Trans fats should be kept to a minimum and avoided altogether when possible.

Chapter 5: Food Groups—Protein and Dairy

Protein and dairy groups are both traditionally dominated by animal-derived foods but have been expanded to include more plant-based foods as our understanding of their nutritional composition has advanced. While the protein food group is the primary source of protein as a macronutrient, both groups contain a wide variety of nutrients. Additionally, these are the food groups most often impacted by non-traditional diet choices such as vegetarian and vegan diets.

What's in the Protein Food Group?

The protein food group consists of foods that are high in protein and has traditionally included meats from cattle, poultry, and other livestock as well as fish and wildlife such as deer. Since the origins of the food pyramid, other high protein foods like nuts, lentils, peas, and beans, some of which are also included in the vegetables food group. Eggs are also part of the proteins food group, though they are often thought of with the dairy food group due to their association with milk.

Dennis Karuri

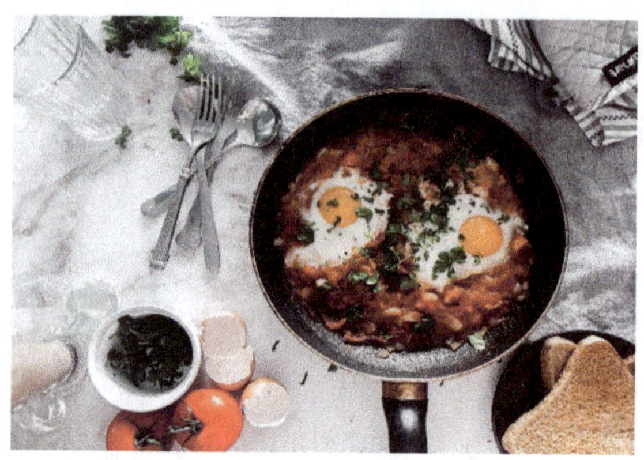

What's in the Dairy Food Group?

The dairy food group consists of animal milk, soymilk, lactose-free milk, and most products that are made from these kinds of milk. This includes ice cream, yogurt, and many kinds of cheese. Notable exclusions from this food group are butter, sour cream, and cream cheese, whose high fat content and low calcium levels put them in the fats and oils food group rather than dairy. Additionally, almond milk and rice milk are not currently considered part of the dairy food group.

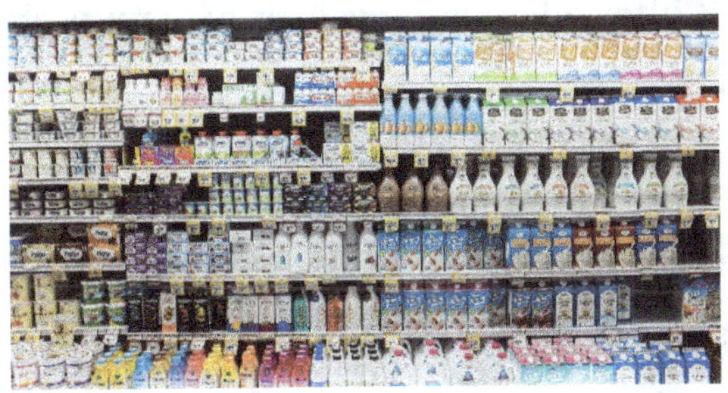

High—Density Nutrients in the Protein Food Group

While all of these foods are high in protein, the types of protein can be more variable which becomes more relevant in certain disease states. Because animal protein profiles are more similar to those of humans, the relative amounts and ratios of amino acids are better balanced to our needs. For generally healthy individuals, however, plants can still offer adequate levels of protein with no ill effects.

In addition to its namesake nutrient, the protein food group is rich in many other nutrients as well. Red meats often contain high levels of iron, as do certain organs such as the liver, and are good sources of B complex vitamins, zinc, and magnesium. High-protein nuts are typically high in many healthy oils, and many kinds of fish are high in omega-3 fatty acids. Vitamin D and vitamin E can also be found in many foods in the protein food group.

Not all of these foods are created equal, though, and some of the foods within the protein groups have a few drawbacks. Many cuts of meat are high in saturated fats, and some fish contain methylmercury which can be toxic at high levels. Care should be taken to select lean meats with little fat and fish with minimal levels of methylmercury.

High—Density Nutrients in the Dairy Food Group

The hallmark of the dairy group is its high calcium levels, but that's not all they have to offer. The different kinds of milk, and a few other products, are often fortified with vitamin D, which goes hand and hand with the appropriate absorption and utilization of calcium. Dairy foods are also a great source of potassium, vitamins A and E along with riboflavin and cobalamin (B12), magnesium, selenium, zinc, and phosphorus. Some products like whole milk also have significant amounts of fat, and many dairy foods provide additional protein and sugars, a form of carbohydrates, to the diet.

Because dairy products are packed with so many kinds of nutrients, they provide a good environment for bacteria to grow. While this is a desirable trait when making products like yogurt, buttermilk, and certain cheeses, it can present a serious threat to human health if left unchecked. To minimize this risk, milk is pasteurized or ultra-pasteurized to minimize the bacterial load before it's shipped to consumers.

This process provides a safer product and helps protect human health, but the high temperatures that destroy the bacteria can also destroy some of milk's nutrients. Many of these can be added back to the final product to restore the nutritional value. Milk and other dairy products should still be refrigerated and periodically checked for freshness as neither pasteurization nor ultra-pasteurization completely removes all the bacteria.

Depending on local regulations, unpasteurized milk, also known as raw milk, may also be available. Unpasteurized milk is often considered to be more nutritionally dense because it isn't subjected to such high temperatures, though there isn't strong support for this theory. The higher levels of bacteria also result in shorter shelf life and an increased risk of food-borne illness. If you include unpasteurized milk in your diet, ensure it is properly stored and handled, and contact a physician at the first sign of illness.

Most soymilk and related products are fortified to provide a similar nutritional profile to traditional dairy products derived from animal milk, providing a healthy option for those choosing non-traditional diets that exclude animal-based dairy products. Almond milk, rice milk, coconut milk, and similar products are often used as replacements for dairy products, but their nutritional profile is rarely comparable to animal milk or fortified soymilk. Those choosing to include these products should consult the nutrition label on the packaging to see what nutrients need to be

Shattering the food pyramid

compensated for in other portions of the diet.

Recommendations for Protein

Similar to grains, recommendations for the protein food group are listed in oz-equiv of protein and are broken into groups by age and gender. Some examples of what constitutes an oz-equiv of protein are one ounce of cooked lean beef or pork, one tablespoon of peanut butter, and one-quarter cup of cooked beans or peas.

Toddlers aged 1 to 2 years old should consume 2 oz-equiv per day while children between 2 and 4 years old need

2 to 5 oz-equiv per day, and children from 5 to 8 should be getting 3 to 5.5 oz-equiv per day. Recommendations for nine years old and up are determined by gender.

Girls from 9 to 13 years old should be getting between 4 and 6 oz-equiv per day, and between 14 and 18 years old, they should get 5 to 6.5 oz-equiv per day. Women should maintain 5 to 6.5 oz-equiv per day from 19 to 30 years old, then decrease slightly to 5 to 6 oz-equiv per day from 31 onward.

Boys from 9 to 13 years old should have 5 to 6.5 oz-equiv per day, and boys from 14 to 18 years old should have 5.5 to 7 oz-equiv per day. Men should consume 6.5 to 7 oz-equiv per day from 19 to 30 years old, then drop their protein intake slightly to 6 to 7 oz-equiv per day between 31 and 59, and decrease again to 5.5 to 6.5 oz-equiv per day from age 60 onward.

Since protein is an essential building block for almost everything within the body, there are times when these recommendations should be increased. Pregnancy is a time when requirements for all nutrients are increased, especially macronutrients like protein. Additionally, protein requirements will increase anytime you're trying to increase muscle mass since it's one of the main constituents of muscle.

Recommendations for

Dairy

Recommendations for dairy are listed in cups, though similar to grains and protein, the amount of a given product that is considered one cup of the dairy food group is variable. For example, milk and yogurt have a 1 to 1 conversion with one cup of these foods also being considered one cup of the dairy food group, but it takes two cups of cottage cheese to get one cup of the dairy food group and two ounces of queso blanco. Dairy food group recommendations are once again broken into age and gender groups.

Toddlers from 1 to 2 years old need 1.5 to 2 cups per day. Children between 2 and 4 years old should get 2 to 2.5 cups per day, and children between 5 and 8 should get 2.5 cups per day.

Unlike grains and proteins, after nine years of age, the recommendations stay the same for all later age and gender groups. Everyone over nine years old should consume 3 cups per day. Dairy requirements increase any time there is an increased need for calcium, most commonly during pregnancy and while breastfeeding for women.

Chapter 6: Food Groups—Fruits and Vegetables

Fruits and vegetables are often considered together, but they have different nutritional profiles and are often consumed in different ways. What makes something a fruit rather than a vegetable is dependent on what context you are considering them in, and some foods are considered vegetables from a dietary and culinary perspective but are considered fruit from a botanical perspective.

What's in the Fruits Food Group?

The fruits food group includes pretty straightforward foods like apples, bananas, kiwis, cantaloupes, and so on. It also includes 100% fruit juices and dried fruits like raisins and prunes. Fruits are often sweet-tasting and can be a healthy snack option. When fresh, they have a high water content that can help you stay hydrated throughout the day.

Dennis Karuri

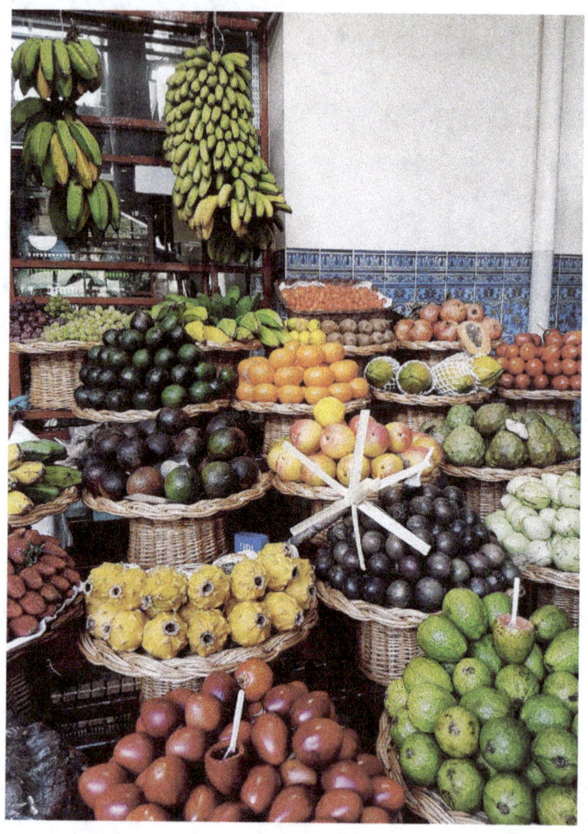

Fruits fall into this category whether they are fresh, cooked, or otherwise processed. They can commonly be found in combination with dairy products in the form of fruit yogurts and smoothies.

Shattering the food pyramid

They can also be cooked into dishes with proteins and are often used in baked desserts like pies and strudels that also include grains.

Many fruit drinks actually contain very little fruit juice and instead have high levels of sweeteners and water with little nutritional value. When looking for drinks to incorporate into the fruits portion of your diet, focus on those specifically stating "100% fruit juice" on the label.

What's in the Vegetables Food Group?

The foods included in the vegetable food group are a little more nuanced and varied than those in the fruit group. The vegetable group is further broken down into dark greens, red and orange vegetables, starchy vegetables, beans, peas, and lentils, and other vegetables. Most vegetables have a more salty or savory flavor than fruits depending on how they're prepared. Vegetables are also more likely to be consumed as sides or cooked into a main dish than eaten alone, though there are a few exceptions to this.

The dark greens category includes spinach, broccoli, and collard greens. Red and orange vegetables include tomatoes, carrots, and sweet potatoes. Starchy vegetables include breadfruit, corn, and plantains. The other vegetables category includes avocados, mushrooms, and onions. The beans, peas, and lentils category has a unique set of characteristics compared to the other vegetable categories.

Beans, peas, and lentils are part of the legume family and are sometimes collectively called pulses. While the term 'legume' refers to the entire plant, pulses are the seed portion that is most commonly consumed. They can also be found in the protein group due to their high protein content. Because of slightly different nutritional profiles, green peas and green lima beans are counted as part of the starchy vegetables category while green, or string, beans are counted as part of the other vegetables category.

Dennis Karuri

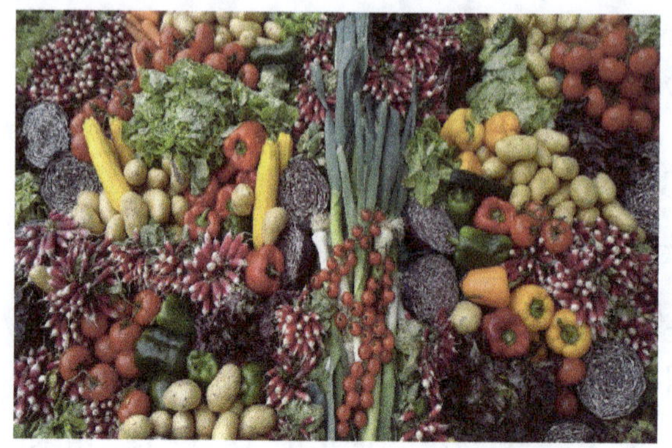

High—Density Nutrients in the Fruits Food Group

The sweet flavors of fruits come from high levels of natural sugars. They are also generally high in micronutrients like vitamin C, potassium, and folate. Fresh and dried fruits are a good source of dietary fiber, though this is absent in fruit juices. The presence of vitamin C aids in the absorption of iron from other parts of the diet, though most fruits don't have significant levels of iron.

Fruits are relatively low calories, have low levels of overall fat, and include no cholesterol. Because they are low in calories but high in fiber, fruits provide a healthy and filling option for snacks and sides. However, because many of the natural sugars are simple sugars, they should still be consumed in moderation.

High—Density Nutrients in the Vegetables Food Group

Vegetables contain a wide variety of nutrients. They are great sources of folate, vitamins A and C, potassium, and dietary fiber. Similar to fruits, vegetable juices lack the fiber content found in whole vegetables. When prepared with minimal sauces and seasonings, vegetables are low in calories and fat, providing a nutrient-dense food that contributes minimally to the overall daily calorie intake. However, many sauces and dressings, like those used to top salads, can add significant fats and calories and should be considered when creating a balanced diet.

Recommendations for Fruits

Recommendations for fruits are measured in cups and can be thought of as on a fresh fruit basis. This means that one cup of fruit or 100% of fruit juice is equal to one cup of the recommended daily intake of the fruit food group, and half a cup of dried fruit, which is more nutrient-dense after the removal of most of the water, is equal to one cup of fresh fruit and, therefore, one cup from the fruit food group. When discussing whole fresh fruit, a little more variability is introduced. One small apple or half of a large apple, ten figs, and eight large strawberries are all equivalent to one cup.

Toddlers aged 1 to 2 years old should consume 0.5 to 1 cup per day. Children between 2 and 4 years old need 1 to 1.5 cups per day, and children from 5 to 8 should be getting 1 to 2 cups per day. Recommendations for nine years old and up vary by gender.

Girls from 9 to 18 years old should be getting between 1.5 to 2 cups per day. Women should maintain 1.5 to 2 cups per day from 19 years onward.

Boys from 9 to 13 years old should get 1.5 to 2 cups per day, and boys from 14 to 18 years old should get 2 to 2.5 cups per day. Men should continue getting 2 to 2.5 cups per day from 19 to 59 years old, then drop to 2 cups per day from age 60 onward.

Recommendations for Vegetables

Vegetable recommendations are also measured in cups. One cup of most raw or cooked vegetables or vegetable juice counts as one cup from the vegetables food group, while two cups of raw leafy greens like those used in salads count as one cup from the vegetable food group. For whole vegetables, some examples of one cup are one large ear of corn, three whole pimentos, five cactus pads, and one medium white potato.

Toddlers aged 1 to 2 years old should consume 0.5 to 1 cup per day. Children between 2 and 4 years old need 1 to 2 cups per day, and children from 5 to 8 should be getting 1.5 to 2.5 cups per day. Recommendations differ based on gender starting at nine years old and up.

Girls from 9 to 13 years old should be getting between 1.5 to 3 cups per day while recommendations for girls between 14 and 18 are 2.5 to 3 cups. Women should maintain 2.5 to 3.5 cups per day from 19 to 30 years old then decrease slightly to 2 to 3 cups per day from age 31 onward.

Boys from 9 to 13 years old should get 2 to 3.5 cups per day, and boys from 14 to 18 years old should get 2.5 to 4 cups per day. Men should have 3 to 4 cups per day from 19 to 59 years old, then drop down to 2.5 to 3.5 cups per day from age 60 onward.

Whether beans, peas, and lentils are considered part of the vegetable food group or the protein food group for any given diet has to do with the relative proportion of other foods from the protein food group. If protein needs are met by consuming meat, poultry, or fish, then pulses can be counted as part of the vegetables food group. If protein needs are not fully met, the pulses can be counted as protein until the recommended amount is reached, then counted as vegetables for any amount over the protein needs.

Chapter 7: Nutrition Gone Awry

While you can't leave out any food group or nutrient entirely, they should all still be included in the diet in moderation. While too little of a nutrient can negatively impact your health, consuming too much creates its own set of concerns as well.

Macronutrient Excesses

While there are some instances where a higher protein diet can be beneficial, consuming higher levels of protein than needed by the body can have detrimental effects. Many times, diets with increased protein have lower levels of carbohydrates and fiber, leading to digestive upset. The increased amounts of protein and lower levels of protein can also push the body into utilizing fat for energy, leading to a build-up of a type of fatty acid called ketones that can eventually reach levels that can have large negative impacts on metabolism and the nervous system.

Excess protein is broken down into its constituent parts, and while the acid group can be shifted into other pathways to be utilized, the amine part is excreted unless the body needs to create more of a specific amino acid. Amines and other nitrogen-containing waste products are excreted through the kidneys.

This increased strain on the kidneys can result in increased thirst and urination, and the increase of these waste products in the blood can cause pH abnormalities, triggering a cascade of events to try to correct the pH problems and increasing the likelihood of kidney stones. If they go on long enough or get severe enough, these changes can cause permanent damage to the kidneys.

Even in more mild cases of protein excess, you can have noticeable changes in breath and body odor. The ketones circulating in the blood can be released in small amounts in the breath, along with some proportion of the nitrogen-containing waste products from the breakdown of protein. The excretion of the remaining nitrogen-containing waste products through the kidneys results in them building up in the urine and carrying an odor.

Fats are incredibly energy-dense, and having excessive fat intake can result in the body increasing the amount it stores. This results in obesity, which can create a strain on the heart and lungs as they try to pump enough blood and take in enough oxygen for the increased body mass.

The increased workload on the heart results in high blood pressure, which in turn increases the risk of heart attack and stroke. This is compounded by higher than normal levels of cholesterol which can form plaques on blood vessel walls, further increasing the strain on the heart.

Increased fats also provide more substrate for the production of hormones and signaling molecules, especially those involved in inflammation. This can lead to chronic, low levels of inflammation triggering a stress response in the body and creating a cascade of effects. These include irregularities in menstrual cycles and decreased fertility for women as well as increased levels of stress hormones that can contribute to feelings of anxiety and irritability and support the mobilization of fat and deposition in abnormal places.

Because carbohydrates are used for energy production, the body will store any carbohydrates consumed in excess of immediate energy demands. This allows for the slow release of glucose to provide energy between meals and compensates for days where intake is insufficient to meet needs. However, carbohydrate intake significantly exceeding energy demands can disrupt the hormonal balance between storage and utilization of energy sources.

Excess consumption can lead to consistently high levels of glucose circulating in the blood, stimulating increased production and release of insulin, the main regulator of glucose levels in the blood. The more insulin cells are exposed to, the more likely they are to become resistant to it, further increasing blood glucose levels as less is driven into the cells to be stored.

This glucose eventually gets taken to the liver, where some of it can be turned into fatty acids and stored for later use. However, continued high blood glucose, called hyperglycemia, results in excessive deposition of fatty acids within the liver and creates what's known as a fatty liver. This build-up of fat takes up a lot of space and eventually starts interfering with the ability of liver cells to function properly.

The effects of insulin and ineffective regulation of blood glucose levels can create a self-perpetuating cycle by causing cravings for carbohydrates, especially sugary sweets, to compensate for the large changes. If allowed to progress long enough, the cells' resistance to insulin and the changes and damage to the liver can become permanent, creating life-long problems.

Macronutrient Deficiencies

While fats are one of the first nutrients to be reduced in many trend and fad diets, inadequate intake can result in deficiencies of important lipids. Fat-soluble vitamins by their very nature need fats to be properly absorbed, leading to further deficiencies. Additionally, while excessive amounts of fat can cause a build-up of fats within arteries, so can deficient amounts of fats because more healthy types of fats help regulate and remove the less healthy fats that are more prone to accumulation.

Omega fatty acids are involved in creating the layers surrounding nerves to protect them and help conduct nerve impulses. A deficiency in fats and lipids means these protective sheaths can't be effectively repaired or replaced. In addition to the potential for nerve damage and degeneration, this deficiency can increase the incidence of mental health disorders like depression, bipolar disorder, and eating disorders.

Protein serves many functions in the body, and inadequate protein intake can affect many systems throughout the body. Most notable is the possibility of muscle wasting as the body breaks down the less important proteins to maintain the production of other types of protein needed to sustain basic functions like the movement of blood, breathing, and nerve function. However, while this can occur with GI diseases preventing the absorption of protein, this is most common in cases of severe malnutrition.

One of protein's many functions is providing oncotic pressure within the blood vessel. When there is inadequate protein to maintain this oncotic pressure where it should be, the fluid leaks out into the tissues, resulting in a condition called edema. Additionally, this balance of fluids between vessels and surrounding tissues helps maintain blood pressure. As protein levels drop, blood pressure can drop, causing light-headedness, faintness, and a decreased heart rate.

Low protein intake also impacts the absorption of micronutrients like zinc, iron, and calcium. As this deficiency goes on, the ability of the body to produce the proteins it needs to maintain the various systems becomes impacted. The immune system begins to lose its function, increasing the risk of infection and disease. Hair begins to thin or fall out and the nails can develop ridges and abnormal growth patterns.

The driving force behind the problems caused by carbohydrate deficiency is the body's need for carbohydrate energy sources, particularly glucose. Red blood cells lack the cellular machinery required to use other energy sources and must use glucose in their metabolism. Many other cells, such as neurons in the brain and immune cells, show an incredible preference for glucose and suffer in its absence.

Because of this preferential utilization of glucose by the brain, one of the first signs of carbohydrate deficiency is low blood sugar, or hypoglycemia, which in turn leads to sluggishness, poor concentration, decreased cognitive performance, and difficulty regulating emotions.

While we do store some reserves in the form of glycogen, those quickly run out, and the body begins to look to fats and proteins to meet its energy demands, though this requires increased intake of these nutrients to compensate, and as discussed in light of protein excess, long-term utilization of fat as a primary energy source can result in the buildup of compounds called ketones.

This is especially true in the case of carbohydrate deficiency because even when fat is mobilized to produce energy, a carbohydrate-derived molecule called oxaloacetate is needed to allow fat to enter the Krebs cycle, also known as the TCA cycle, to generate energy and spare glucose for the cells that need it the most. As this runs out, ketones begin to accumulate even faster because there's no good way to use them.

When the body runs out of carbohydrates and risks running out of glucose, it begins breaking down proteins and utilizing amino acids for their carbon backbone. The amino acids glutamate and alanine can be converted directly into glucose, but the remaining amino acids must be further broken down, introduced into the Krebs cycle, and converted into other molecules that can exit the Krebs cycle and become glucose.

However, unless there is sufficient protein intake to match the energy demands of the body, this process has very limited utility because the body can only mobilize and break down so much protein from muscle. This can result in an inability to maintain necessary amounts of glucose to allow for proper function and increases the risk of a high level of ketones that can produce toxic effects, including neurologic and behavioral changes. Even in cases where protein intake can meet energy demands, you still have to consider the concerns brought up by excessive protein intake.

Micronutrient Excesses

Excess amounts of iron, typically from overconsumption of iron supplements, result in predominantly GI symptoms, including abdominal pain, liver damage, and low blood sugar. These can lead to shock, seizure, and even coma, eventually resulting in death if not successfully treated.

Zinc toxicity manifests as general symptoms of nausea, vomiting, and diarrhea. Excess zinc prevents proper absorption of copper. It can also cause damage to the nervous system along with the rupture and destruction of red blood cells.

Copper excess causes problems primarily by accumulating at high levels in various organs, including the brain, liver, kidneys, and most other organs. This accumulation can lead to neurologic deficits, liver failure, kidney failure, and dysfunction of whatever organ the accumulation is found in.

Calcium and phosphorus are closely related minerals, and an excess of one can trigger a deficiency in the other because of the way they are coregulated. Additionally, because they can bind and complex together, they can deposit within various tissues whenever either of them is in excess.

The symptoms of iodine excess are typically the result of subsequent overproduction of thyroid hormone. This is a form of hyperthyroidism and causes metabolism-driven problems like weight loss and increased BP/HR, and can lead to feelings of anxiety. Selenium excess starts with non-specific signs like nausea and weakness. As selenium builds up, it can cause brittle hair and nails as well as damage to the nerves and how it functions.

Sodium is maintained in a very narrow window by the body, and an excess interferes with nerve conduction, which can trigger seizures and convulsions. It also pulls water out of cells, especially those within the brain, and a rapid correction of excess sodium can lead to brain damage as water rushes back into the cells.

Potassium is less tightly regulated than sodium. However, it is still very sensitive to excesses, and the body will try to regulate the level of circulating potassium by driving it into cells and vomiting when high levels are consumed. Excesses are still possible, though, and this can lead to cardiac arrhythmia and arrest due to overexcitement of the muscle cells in the heart.

While minerals are often the first thing to come to mind when thinking about micronutrient excesses, vitamins can also be consumed in enough amounts to cause toxicity. Fat-soluble vitamins are more often found in excess than water-soluble because of the way the body stores them.

Vitamin A excesses lead to the drying out of mucous membranes on the inside the nose and lining the eyelids and can increase the pressure within the skull, causing headaches and nausea. In children, there can be pain and inflammation of the bones, and dry, itchy skin with hair loss can occur in both adults and children.

Pyridoxine excess only has detrimental effects at very high doses, and these typically include damage to nerves that manifests as changes to walking and superficial loss of sensation with loss of spatial awareness and coordination occurring at incredibly massive levels of excess.

Niacin excess has mild effects at small excesses such as dilation of the blood vessels and flushing of the skin as capillaries open up. However, as the levels increase, there can be increased vessel dilation, headaches, nausea, and occasional problems with the skin. If excesses are maintained over long periods of time, insulin resistance can occur, along with subsequent mobilization of fat.

Vitamin C is relatively non-toxic in excess, with some GI symptoms at very high levels. There is some concern over other potential impacts, but none have been supported by research.

Excess vitamin D greatly impacts calcium metabolism and regulation and can result in excessive levels of calcium being absorbed from the intestines and being pulled out of bones with a resultant low phosphorus level. This results in softer, weaker bones with deposition of calcium in soft tissues.

Micronutrient Deficiencies

While micronutrient deficiencies are often studied in the context of children and pregnant women due to their key role in growth and development, they can occur in anyone with an inadequate or unbalanced diet. However, the problems caused by these deficiencies can vary between different age groups.

Iron deficiency leads to anemia and an impaired ability to transport oxygen in the blood to the various tissues. In addition to inadequate intake, iron deficiency is seen after blood loss, such as from a traumatic injury, and is common at a mild, subclinical level in menstruating women.

A deficiency of zinc means impairment of all of its functions, especially those in the immune system. The ability of the skin to prevent bacteria and other disease-causing organisms begins to fail, and the immune system can no longer effectively fight off these invaders. Because of its role in cell division, zinc deficiency can also slow growth. Hair loss and impaired sight, taste, and smell are other signs of increasing degrees of deficiency.

Like many micronutrients, the effects of a selenium deficiency are most pronounced in children, resulting in oxidative damage to the growing muscles that causes weakness. If severe enough, it can impact the muscles of the heart, leading to heart failure and eventual death. Selenium deficiency can also have a negative impact on immune function, and the reduction in the body's antioxidant capabilities can result in accumulated cell damage from the natural byproducts of metabolism.

Because calcium is vital to the strength and integrity of bones, a deficiency leads to weak, almost soft bone seen as Rickets in children and as osteomalacia, a nutritionally-based weakening of the bones, or osteoporosis, the decrease of the amount of bone over time. A calcium deficiency, also called hypocalcemia, can also lead to muscle weakness because muscles are unable to properly contract without enough calcium.

Magnesium deficiency can also result in muscle weakness by interfering with the nerve signals to the muscle, and through a similar mechanism, it can interfere with conduction and signaling in the brain, resulting in a lack of energy and, sometimes, behavior and attitude changes. If severe enough for an extended period of time, the impacts of low magnesium can lead to rigid muscles and seizures, though it can often be caught and treated before this point.

Potassium deficiency can manifest as muscle fatigue and weakness, high blood pressure, and tingling or numbness. An inadequate amount of potassium in the nerve cells reduces their ability to transmit information, and in the heart, it can lead to an inability to contract properly, leading to a backup of blood and eventual heart failure. Potassium is also essential in maintaining blood pH, and deficiency can lead to a host of acid-base disturbances with wide-ranging impacts.

Calcium, magnesium, and potassium deficiencies are often concurrent problems. Their symptoms can appear to be overlapping, and distinguishing them often requires blood tests.

Iodine is closely tied to thyroid function, and a deficiency can have a wide range of symptoms that mirror thyroid problems. Inadequate thyroid function or even thyroid failure can be seen, and a birth defect known as cretinism is common when women are severely deficient during pregnancy. During childhood, an iodine deficiency can lead to delayed growth and brain damage, while in adults the most common signs are loss of energy, weight gain, and hair loss. Goiter is a variable presentation and can be seen at any age.

Deficiencies in vitamins have the same kind of variability as excesses, though the prevalence tends to be reversed between fat-soluble and water-soluble vitamins, at least in adults, because the body can create larger stores of fat-soluble vitamins while they're abundant to use when they become scarce.

An important though uncommon vitamin deficiency is vitamin K deficiency, which, in addition to dietary inadequacy, can be induced by accidental ingestion of some rat poisons or an overdose of certain medications like warfarin. Vitamin K deficiency results in an inability to properly form a clot and if severe enough, can lead to uncontrolled bleeding throughout the body, commonly identified by petechiae, ecchymoses, and a loss of energy or collapse due to the loss of blood from vessels.

A mild vitamin A deficiency can be difficult to detect, but it can have significant consequences even without overt signs. It's most prominent in children where it causes night blindness and malformations and damage to the cornea that can progress to complete blindness as well as a higher incidence and severity of infectious diseases. Deficiency can also delay growth, lead to anemia as the production of red blood cells is impaired, and alters the types of cells found in mucosal surfaces like those in the lungs, reducing the function of those surfaces and their ability to fend off infection.

Thiamine (B1) deficiency can lead to a condition called beriberi, a disease characterized by damage to the nervous system resulting in tingling sensations and weakness, heart disease with an abnormally increased and visible pulse in the jugular vein and an increased difference between systolic and diastolic blood pressure, and edema throughout the body.

Riboflavin deficiency is rarely seen alone due to its coexistence with many other nutrients, but it leads to widespread, chronic inflammation. This is seen as ulcers of the mouth and tongue, anemia, light sensitivity, and scaly irritation of the skin on the face.

Inadequate niacin also causes scaly irritation of the skin, though, with this vitamin, the irritation is focused on parts of the body exposed to pressure, like the knees and elbows, or sunlight. On top of the skin irritation, the cells lining the intestines wither and shrink, and there can be decreased amounts of the hormone serotonin produced in the brain, leading to dementia.

A deficiency of folate causes a form of anemia characterized by large, immature red blood cells as well as congenital defects involving the brain and spinal cord. Cobalamin, following the trend set by niacin and riboflavin, also causes anemia, this time featuring red blood cells that are large but fully matured, and can lead to severe neurological problems including a loss of coordination of voluntary movements, dementia, and memory loss.

Vitamin D's role in homeostasis means a deficiency leads to a wide array of symptoms from high blood pressure to calcium deficiency. It also leads to decreased immune function, and because of the resultant hypocalcemia, you can see things like rickets and osteomalacia even when calcium in the diet is adequate. The calcium imbalance can also trigger a secondarily overactive parathyroid gland that can cause excessive excretion of phosphorus in an effort to correct hypocalcemia.

A lack of vitamin C leads to weakened and improperly formed connective tissue, known as scurvy, and a general feeling of weakness and fatigue. Because connective tissue can't be properly formed, there is often a lack of adequate healing, and its role in iron absorption can predispose to an iron deficiency.

Vitamin E deficiency has similar effects to selenium deficiency due to their interrelated antioxidant functions. In children, it manifests as loss of coordination and spatial awareness, muscle weakness, and difficulty walking while adults rarely have a significant enough deficiency to show signs. It can also lead to the rupture of red blood cells within the vessels at any age.

Conclusion

Nutrition is a complex yet essential subject that is a core principle in maintaining overall health. Governments, along with some educational institutes and health organizations, have made an effort to make nutritional guidance available to all.

The basics of nutrition can be broken into macronutrients, those needed in larger quantities, and micronutrients, those needed in smaller amounts. Macronutrients and micronutrients are what actually needs to be considered when creating a balanced diet, and the recommendations for the different food groups are based on relative levels of these nutrients.

Macronutrients are carbohydrates, proteins, and fats, all of which are complex molecules that can take on a variety of different forms. They are the main drivers of energy and calorie intake, and they act as the main building blocks of the body.

Micronutrients consist of vitamins and minerals. Six different groups of vitamins and more than a dozen minerals are needed by the body. They act as cofactors for reactions throughout the body and support the function of different body systems like the nervous and musculoskeletal systems.

Each nutrient fulfills numerous functions, and many of them act synergistically with each other. No one food contains adequate amounts of all of them without also providing excessive amounts of others. A variety of different kinds of foods, even within a given food group, is needed to get the right amount of everything without excess or deficiency.

The six major food groups are grains, protein, dairy, fruits, vegetables, and fats and oils. Each group has its own unique characteristics and attributes as well as different predominant nutrients. While every food within a group will have different amounts of these nutrients, recommendations for daily intake of each group can be made as long as a variety of foods within the group are included.

Non-traditional diets such as dairy-free, gluten-free, and vegan or vegetarian, can still meet nutritional needs as long as care is taken to include all the necessary nutrients. Certain vegetables, for example, can provide an alternative protein source to meet, and soy products can be fortified to provide all the same nutrients as animal milk.

There is no universal amount of any nutrient that is perfect for everyone. However, some general recommendations can be made for broad groups of people based on a handful of characteristics, typically age and gender, and provide a good starting point for creating a balanced diet. These recommendations don't take into account all factors and should be modified to account for activity level, pregnancy or lactation, and health status, among other things.

Every nutrient should be consumed in moderation, and a deficiency or excess of any of them can have deleterious effects. Efforts should be made to create a balanced diet to ensure adequate nutrient intake and support health and well-being.

The recommendations seen on graphics like food pyramids and food plates provide a good starting point, but they need to be tailored to an individual's specific circumstances. With this knowledge, you have a foundation to better utilize the information available to create a balanced diet and start the journey to becoming your best self.

Glossary

Amphipathic: a molecule with a hydrophobic and a hydrophilic portion

Balanced Diet: a diet that provides all macronutrients and micronutrients at levels that meet the needs of the body with little excess

Bioavailability: the amount of a nutrient, usually vitamins and minerals, that can be absorbed and is available to be utilized by the body

Bran: the outer seed coats of grains that are broken and sifted out of refined flours and meals

Calorie: the amount of energy required to raise the temperature of 1 gram of water $1^{\circ}C$; in nutrition, refers to a kilocalorie and is used to measure the energy in food

Calorimeter: a device used to measure the number of calories in a material by placing it in a chamber submerged in water and igniting it

Catalyze: to initiate or accelerate a chemical reaction

Cell Turnover: a natural, continuous process in which cells reach the end of their lifespan, die and are replaced by new cells of the same type

Coagulation Cascade: a series of reactions within the body to form a clot to seal a blood vessel and stop bleeding

Cofactors: molecules needed to activate enzymes and allow reactions to proceed

Cognitive: involving the ability to use conscious, intellectual ability, reasoning, and thinking

Ecchymoses: large areas of blood pooling under the skin, commonly due to an inability to clot properly and seal small imperfections created in capillaries; not to be confused with bruising that is caused by the sudden, traumatic rupture of capillaries below the skin

Edema: the accumulation of fluid outside blood vessels in the space between cells

Endosperm: the nutrient-dense portion of seeds and grains that supports the growth of the plant

Enriched Bread: bread made with enriched flour; see *enriched flour*

Enriched Flour: flour with added vitamins and minerals to replace those lost during the milling process to turn wheat into flour

Esterification: a reaction between an acid and alcohol that creates an ester

Fortified Milk: milk with vitamins A and D added to replace those destroyed by the high heat during the pasteurization process

Gluconeogenesis: the process of using lactate, proteins, and glycerol to create new molecules of glucose for the body to use as an energy source when carbohydrate sources of glucose are insufficient

Germ: the part of seeds and grains that sprouts and grows into a plant

Hydrogenation: the process of adding hydrogen atoms to unsaturated fats to reduce the number of double bonds between carbon atoms, creating trans fatty acids

Hydrophilic: able to mix with or dissolve in water

Hydrophobic: able to repel or remain separate from water

Kilocalorie: 1,000 calories, written as kcals and sometimes as Calories

Non-covalent Bonds: a form of molecular bonding that results from electromagnetic attraction rather than the sharing of electrons

Oncotic Pressure: the influence of molecules within a vessel that pulls fluids into the vessel from surrounding tissue

Pasteurize: a process used to reduce bacterial loads in many products, including milk and fruit juices; heating a liquid to 161°F (72°C) for a minimum of 15 seconds then packaging in clean, sanitized conditions

Petechiae: small, pinpoint spots of bleeding below the skin caused by a deficiency in the coagulation cascade's ability to form clots

Staple Foods: foods that make up a large portion of the diets of a given population; these vary greatly by region and culture

Ultra-pasteurized: a form of pasteurization utilizing higher temperatures for shorter times; heating a liquid to 280°F (138°C) for a minimum of 2 seconds then packaging it in nearly sterile conditions

References

Bharati, K. (2017, March 10). *Mineral deficiency - What should you know?* Medindia. https://www.medindia.net/patie ntinfo/mineral-deficiency.htm

Brusie, C. (2017, October 3). *How did the government get the food pyramid so terribly wrong?* HealthyWay. https://www.healthyway.com/co ntent/how-did-the-government-get-the-food-pyramid-so-terribly-wrong/

Cleveland Clinic. (2014, November 28). *Healthy Fat Intake.* Cleveland Clinic. https://my.clevelandclinic.org/he

alth/articles/11208-fat-what-you-need-to-know#:~:text=The%20dietary%20oreference%20intake%20

Combs, G. F., & McClung, J. P. (2017). *Chapter 5 - Vitamin Needs and Safety*. (G. F. Combs & J. P. McClung Eds.). The Vitamins (Fifth Edition) Fundamental Aspects in Nutrition and Health (pp. 79–106). Academic Press. https://reader.elsevier.com/reader/sd/pii/B9780128029657000058?token=3CC95D864A2DB70A946E458654A7C1C06E5D1AB9650B6EB76775A9034A7BBEC15437FDA9E38F594965FC75275A263F09&originRegion=us-east-1&originCreation=20220412021710

Cornell University. (2007). *Pasteurized versus Ultra-Pasteurized Milk - Why Such Long Sell-By Dates?* https://foodsafety.foodscience.co rnell.edu/sites/foodsafety.foodsci ence.cornell.edu/files/shared/do cuments/CU-DFScience-Notes-Milk-Pasteurization-UltraP-10-10.pdf

Extension Nutrition and Wellness Specialist, Department of Extension Family and Consumer Sciences, New Mexico State University. (2018, November). *NMSU: MyPlate - The fruit group: Focus on fruits.* Aces.nmsu.edu. https://aces.nmsu.edu/pubs/_e/ E141/welcome.html

Dennis Karuri

FDA Center for Food Safety. (2020, May 5). *Daily value on the new nutrition and supplement facts labels.* FDA. https://www.fda.gov/food/new-nutrition-facts-label/daily-value-new-nutrition-and-supplement-facts-labels

Food and Agriculture Organization of the United Nations. (n.d.). *Food-based dietary guidelines - United Kingdom.* Food and Agriculture Organization of the United Nations. https://www.fao.org/nutrition/education/food-dietary-guidelines/regions/countries/united-kingdom/en/

Griffiths, J. K. (2013). *139 - Vitamin Deficiencies.* (A. J. Magill, D. R.

Hill, T. Solomon, & E. T. Ryan Eds.). Hunter's Tropical Medicine and Emerging Infectious Disease (Ninth Edition) (pp. 997–1002). W.B. Saunders. https://www.sciencedirect.com/science/article/pii/B9781416043904001399

Hanson, R. W., & Owen, O. E. (2013). *Gluconeogenesis.* (W. J. Lamarz & M. D. Lane Eds.). Encyclopedia of Biological Chemistry (2nd ed., pp. 381–386). Academic Press. https://reader.elsevier.com/reader/sd/pii/B978012378630200040 2?token=EE90EED3ADE216D7 BBCB5501F484449589989B472 068263D4702C4B09527A2BE0F 1E155B7FCAED267A88B1139F24 2F49&originRegion=us-east-

1&originCreation=202204062312
34

Harvard Health Publishing. (2017,
August 14). *Listing of vitamins.*
Harvard Health; Harvard Health.
https://www.health.harvard.edu/
staying-
healthy/listing_of_vitamins

Harvard School of Public Health. (2018,
July 24). *Types of fat.* The
Nutrition   Source.
https://www.hsph.harvard.edu/n
utritionsource/what-should-you-
eat/fats-and-cholesterol/types-
of-fat/

Harvard School of Public Health. (2019).
Healthy eating plate. The
Nutrition   Source.
https://www.hsph.harvard.edu/n

utritionsource/healthy-eating-plate/

Johnson, L. E. (2020, November). *Vitamin E deficiency - Disorders of nutrition*. Merck Manuals Consumer Version. https://www.merckmanuals.com/home/disorders-of-nutrition/vitamins/vitamin-e-deficiency

Kubala, J. (2022, February 3). *Essential amino acids: Definition, benefits and food sources*. Healthline. https://www.healthline.com/nutrition/essential-amino-acids#what-they-are

McLeod, H. (2021, March 25). *A history of the food pyramid*. Smokymountainnews.com. https://smokymountainnews.co

m/lifestyle/rumble/item/31055-
a-history-of-the-food-pyramid

*Mineral Toxicity - symptoms, meaning,
Definition, Description,
Demographics, Causes and
symptoms, Diagnosis.* (2013). In
Encyclopedia of Children's
Health.
http://www.healthofchildren.co
m/M/Mineral-Toxicity.html

National Institutes of Health. (2017a).
*Office of dietary supplements -
Folate.* Nih.gov.
https://ods.od.nih.gov/factsheets
/Folate-HealthProfessional/

National Institutes of Health. (2017b).
*Office of dietary supplements -
Manganese.* Nih.gov.
https://ods.od.nih.gov/factsheets
/Manganese-HealthProfessional/

Nature Education. (2010). *Protein structure.* Nature.com. https://www.nature.com/scitable /topicpage/protein-structure-14122136/

New Skills Academy. (n.d.). Module 3 - Macronutrients in Food: Proteins, Fats, and Carbohydrates (Part I). [MOOC lecture]. *Introduction to Nutrition Certification.* New Skills Academy. https://newskillsacademy.com/c ourse/introduction-nutrition-certification

New Skills Academy. (n.d.). Module 4 - Macronutrients in Food: Proteins, Fats, and Carbohydrates (Part II). [MOOC lecture]. *Introduction to*

Nutrition Certification. New Skills Academy. https://newskillsacademy.com/course/introduction-nutrition-certification

New Skills Academy. (n.d.). Module 5 - Digestion and Metabolism of Fats and Micronutrients, and their Role in Nutrition (I). [MOOC lecture]. *Introduction to Nutrition Certification.* New Skills Academy. https://newskillsacademy.com/course/introduction-nutrition-certification

New Skills Academy. (n.d.). Module 6 - Micronutrients, and their Role in Nutrition (II). [MOOC lecture]. *Introduction to*

Nutrition Certification. New Skills Academy. https://newskillsacademy.com/course/introduction-nutrition-certification

New Skills Academy. (n.d.). Module 7 -Micronutrients, and their Role in Nutrition (III) (Vitamin B Complex, Minerals, and Electrolytes). [MOOC lecture]. *Introduction to Nutrition Certification*. New Skills Academy. https://newskillsacademy.com/course/introduction-nutrition-certification

Public Health England. (2016). *From plate to guide: What, why and how for the eatwell model.* https://assets.publishing.service.

gov.uk/government/uploads/syst
em/uploads/attachment_data/fil
e/579388/eatwell_model_guide
_report.pdf

Scott. (2013, February 15). *Fact or myth: Sodium raises blood pressure*. Today I Found Out. http://www.todayifoundout.com/index.php/2013/02/why-does-salt-raise-blood-pressure/

Shankar, A. H. (2013). *140 - Mineral Deficiencies*. (A. J. Magill, D. R. Hill, T. Solomon, & E. T. Ryan, Eds.). Hunter's Tropical Medicine and Emerging Infectious Disease (Ninth Edition) (pp. 1003–1010). W.B. Saunders. https://www.sciencedirect.com/science/article/pii/B9781416043904001405

Smallwood, K. (2014, August 24). *Who invented the food pyramid?* Today I Found Out. http://www.todayifoundout.com/index.php/2013/09/invented-food-pyramid/

Spritzler, F. (2020, October 5). *Fat grams: How much fat should you eat per day?* Healthline. https://www.healthline.com/nutrition/how-much-fat-to-eat#TOC_TITLE_HDR_5

USDA. (2020a). *Beans, peas, and lentils.* Myplate.gov. https://www.myplate.gov/eat-healthy/protein-foods/beans-and-peas

USDA. (2020b). *Dairy.* Myplate.gov. https://www.myplate.gov/eat-healthy/dairy

USDA. (2020c). *Fruits*. Myplate.gov.
https://www.myplate.gov/eat-healthy/fruits

USDA. (2020d). Grains. Myplate.gov.
https://www.myplate.gov/eat-healthy/grains

USDA. (2020e). *Protein foods*. Myplate.gov.
https://www.myplate.gov/eat-healthy/protein-foods

USDA. (2020f). *Vegetables*. Myplate.gov.
https://www.myplate.gov/eat-healthy/vegetables

USDHHS ODPHP. (2020, December 29). *Appendix E-3.6*. Health.gov.
https://health.gov/our-work/nutrition-physical-activity/dietary-guidelines/previous-dietary-

guidelines/2015/advisory-report/appendix-e-3/appendix-e-36

White, B. (2009). Dietary Fatty Acids. *American Family Physician*, 80(4), 345–350. https://www.aafp.org/afp/2009/0815/p345.html

Image References

dandelion_tea. (2020, June 22). *Food pyramid*. [ClipArt]. Pixabay.com. https://pixabay.com/vectors/food-pyramid-eating-pyramid-5329204/

Du Preez, P. (2016, September 27). *Whole grain muffins with head of wheat*. [Photograph]. Unsplash.com.

Dennis Karuri

https://unsplash.com/photos/LRKvds1j
f1Q

Eliason, K. (2017, September 28). *Grocery store dairy section.* [Photograph]. Unsplash.com. https://unsplash.com/photos/SvhXD3k PSTY

Garnier, C. (2019, August 21). *Mix of vegetables at the flower show in Chantilly.* [Photograph]. Unsplash.com. https://unsplash.com/photos/910Ganw Boew

NB, M. (2021, February 28). *Shakshuka eggs for breakfast.* [Photograph]. Unsplash.com. https://unsplash.com/photos/KD93b4X evCQ

OpenClipart-Vectors. (2013, October 15). *DNA amino acids circle graph.* [Infographic]. Pixabay.com.

https://pixabay.com/vectors/dna-amino-acids-biology-code-152136/

Reiseuhu. (2019, June 17). *Assorted fruits on display.* [Photograph]. Unsplash.com. https://unsplash.com/photos/JI5VdAD2mAo

Sinigersky, A. (2018, June 6). *Assorted labeled bottle on display shelf.* [Photograph]. Unsplash.com. https://unsplash.com/photos/THdmJFIBEI8

Sorge, R. (2016, September 27). *Olive oil.* [Photograph]. Unsplash.com. https://unsplash.com/photos/uOBApnN_K7w

Spratt, A. (2018, July 21). *Vintage page containing food groups.* [Photograph]. Unsplash.com.

Dennis Karuri

https://unsplash.com/photos/Xwb1Xp
N7nEQ